Monitoring Blood Sugar - for Men

ISBN-13: 978-1539021865
ISBN-10: 1539021866

First Printing - 2016

Manufactured in the United States of America

Monitoring Blood Sugar - for Men

The purpose of this Blood Sugar Log is threefold:

- Know how your blood sugar varies over time after eating
- Pinpoint what foods spike your blood sugar
- Pinpoint how much food causes a spike in your blood sugar

This log works for whatever monitoring schedule you choose, whether it be every meal or whenever it is convenient to take your reading.

At some point in your logging you will begin to see patterns, and that will allow you to adjust the kinds of foods and the specific portion size changes to have the greatest reduction in blood sugar spiking with the least inconvenience

Date:		Reading Before	Reading 1 hr After	Reading 2 hrs After	Reading 4 hrs After
Which Meal:					
Time Start:					
Time End:					
What I Ate and How Much					
Comments :					

Date:		Reading Before	Reading 1 hr After	Reading 2 hrs After	Reading 4 hrs After
Which Meal:					
Time Start:					
Time End:					
What I Ate and How Much					
Comments :					

Date:		Reading Before	Reading 1 hr After	Reading 2 hrs After	Reading 4 hrs After
Which Meal:					
Time Start:					
Time End:					
What I Ate and How Much					
Comments :					

Date:		Reading Before	Reading 1 hr After	Reading 2 hrs After	Reading 4 hrs After
Which Meal:					
Time Start:					
Time End:					
What I Ate and How Much					
Comments :					

Date:		Reading Before	Reading 1 hr After	Reading 2 hrs After	Reading 4 hrs After
Which Meal:					
Time Start:					
Time End:					
What I Ate and How Much					
Comments :					

Date:		Reading Before	Reading 1 hr After	Reading 2 hrs After	Reading 4 hrs After
Which Meal:					
Time Start:					
Time End:					
What I Ate and How Much					
Comments :					

Date:		Reading Before	Reading 1 hr After	Reading 2 hrs After	Reading 4 hrs After
Which Meal:					
Time Start:					
Time End:					
What I Ate and How Much					
Comments :					

Date:		Reading Before	Reading 1 hr After	Reading 2 hrs After	Reading 4 hrs After
Which Meal:					
Time Start:					
Time End:					
What I Ate and How Much					
Comments :					

Date:		Reading Before	Reading 1 hr After	Reading 2 hrs After	Reading 4 hrs After
Which Meal:					
Time Start:					
Time End:					
What I Ate and How Much					
Comments :					

Date:		Reading Before	Reading 1 hr After	Reading 2 hrs After	Reading 4 hrs After
Which Meal:					
Time Start:					
Time End:					
What I Ate and How Much					
Comments :					

Date:		Reading Before	Reading 1 hr After	Reading 2 hrs After	Reading 4 hrs After
Which Meal:					
Time Start:					
Time End:					
What I Ate and How Much					
Comments :					

Date:		Reading Before	Reading 1 hr After	Reading 2 hrs After	Reading 4 hrs After
Which Meal:					
Time Start:					
Time End:					
What I Ate and How Much					
Comments :					

Date:		Reading Before	Reading 1 hr After	Reading 2 hrs After	Reading 4 hrs After
Which Meal:					
Time Start:					
Time End:					
What I Ate and How Much					
Comments :					

Date:		Reading Before	Reading 1 hr After	Reading 2 hrs After	Reading 4 hrs After
Which Meal:					
Time Start:					
Time End:					
What I Ate and How Much					
Comments :					

Date:		Reading Before	Reading 1 hr After	Reading 2 hrs After	Reading 4 hrs After
Which Meal:					
Time Start:					
Time End:					
What I Ate and How Much					
Comments :					

Date:		Reading Before	Reading 1 hr After	Reading 2 hrs After	Reading 4 hrs After
Which Meal:					
Time Start:					
Time End:					
What I Ate and How Much					
Comments :					

Date:		Reading Before	Reading 1 hr After	Reading 2 hrs After	Reading 4 hrs After
Which Meal:					
Time Start:					
Time End:					
What I Ate and How Much					
Comments :					

Date:		Reading Before	Reading 1 hr After	Reading 2 hrs After	Reading 4 hrs After
Which Meal:					
Time Start:					
Time End:					
What I Ate and How Much					
Comments :					

Date:		Reading Before	Reading 1 hr After	Reading 2 hrs After	Reading 4 hrs After
Which Meal:					
Time Start:					
Time End:					
What I Ate and How Much					
Comments:					

Date:		Reading Before	Reading 1 hr After	Reading 2 hrs After	Reading 4 hrs After
Which Meal:					
Time Start:					
Time End:					
What I Ate and How Much					
Comments:					

Date:		Reading Before	Reading 1 hr After	Reading 2 hrs After	Reading 4 hrs After
Which Meal:					
Time Start:					
Time End:					
What I Ate and How Much					
Comments:					

Date:		Reading Before	Reading 1 hr After	Reading 2 hrs After	Reading 4 hrs After
Which Meal:					
Time Start:					
Time End:					
What I Ate and How Much					
Comments :					

Date:		Reading Before	Reading 1 hr After	Reading 2 hrs After	Reading 4 hrs After
Which Meal:					
Time Start:					
Time End:					
What I Ate and How Much					
Comments :					

Date:		Reading Before	Reading 1 hr After	Reading 2 hrs After	Reading 4 hrs After
Which Meal:					
Time Start:					
Time End:					
What I Ate and How Much					
Comments :					

Date:		Reading Before	Reading 1 hr After	Reading 2 hrs After	Reading 4 hrs After
Which Meal:					
Time Start:					
Time End:					
What I Ate and How Much					
Comments:					

Date:		Reading Before	Reading 1 hr After	Reading 2 hrs After	Reading 4 hrs After
Which Meal:					
Time Start:					
Time End:					
What I Ate and How Much					
Comments:					

Date:		Reading Before	Reading 1 hr After	Reading 2 hrs After	Reading 4 hrs After
Which Meal:					
Time Start:					
Time End:					
What I Ate and How Much					
Comments:					

Date:		Reading Before	Reading 1 hr After	Reading 2 hrs After	Reading 4 hrs After
Which Meal:					
Time Start:					
Time End					
What I Ate and How Much					
Comments :					

Date:		Reading Before	Reading 1 hr After	Reading 2 hrs After	Reading 4 hrs After
Which Meal:					
Time Start:					
Time End:					
What I Ate and How Much					
Comments :					

Date:		Reading Before	Reading 1 hr After	Reading 2 hrs After	Reading 4 hrs After
Which Meal:					
Time Start:					
Time End:					
What I Ate and How Much					
Comments :					

Date:		Reading Before	Reading 1 hr After	Reading 2 hrs After	Reading 4 hrs After
Which Meal:					
Time Start:					
Time End:					
What I Ate and How Much					
Comments :					

Date:		Reading Before	Reading 1 hr After	Reading 2 hrs After	Reading 4 hrs After
Which Meal:					
Time Start:					
Time End:					
What I Ate and How Much					
Comments :					

Date:		Reading Before	Reading 1 hr After	Reading 2 hrs After	Reading 4 hrs After
Which Meal:					
Time Start:					
Time End:					
What I Ate and How Much					
Comments :					

Date:		Reading Before	Reading 1 hr After	Reading 2 hrs After	Reading 4 hrs After
Which Meal:					
Time Start:					
Time End:					
What I Ate and How Much					
Comments:					

Date:		Reading Before	Reading 1 hr After	Reading 2 hrs After	Reading 4 hrs After
Which Meal:					
Time Start:					
Time End:					
What I Ate and How Much					
Comments:					

Date:		Reading Before	Reading 1 hr After	Reading 2 hrs After	Reading 4 hrs After
Which Meal:					
Time Start:					
Time End:					
What I Ate and How Much					
Comments:					

Date:		Reading Before	Reading 1 hr After	Reading 2 hrs After	Reading 4 hrs After
Which Meal:					
Time Start:					
Time End:					
What I Ate and How Much					
Comments :					

Date:		Reading Before	Reading 1 hr After	Reading 2 hrs After	Reading 4 hrs After
Which Meal:					
Time Start:					
Time End:					
What I Ate and How Much					
Comments :					

Date:		Reading Before	Reading 1 hr After	Reading 2 hrs After	Reading 4 hrs After
Which Meal:					
Time Start:					
Time End:					
What I Ate and How Much					
Comments :					

Date:		Reading Before	Reading 1 hr After	Reading 2 hrs After	Reading 4 hrs After
Which Meal:					
Time Start:					
Time End:					
What I Ate and How Much					
Comments :					

Date:		Reading Before	Reading 1 hr After	Reading 2 hrs After	Reading 4 hrs After
Which Meal:					
Time Start:					
Time End:					
What I Ate and How Much					
Comments :					

Date:		Reading Before	Reading 1 hr After	Reading 2 hrs After	Reading 4 hrs After
Which Meal:					
Time Start:					
Time End:					
What I Ate and How Much					
Comments :					

Date:		Reading Before	Reading 1 hr After	Reading 2 hrs After	Reading 4 hrs After
Which Meal:					
Time Start:					
Time End:					
What I Ate and How Much					
Comments :					

Date:		Reading Before	Reading 1 hr After	Reading 2 hrs After	Reading 4 hrs After
Which Meal:					
Time Start:					
Time End:					
What I Ate and How Much					
Comments :					

Date:		Reading Before	Reading 1 hr After	Reading 2 hrs After	Reading 4 hrs After
Which Meal:					
Time Start:					
Time End:					
What I Ate and How Much					
Comments :					

Date:		Reading Before	Reading 1 hr After	Reading 2 hrs After	Reading 4 hrs After
Which Meal:					
Time Start:					
Time End:					
What I Ate and How Much					
Comments :					

Date:		Reading Before	Reading 1 hr After	Reading 2 hrs After	Reading 4 hrs After
Which Meal:					
Time Start:					
Time End:					
What I Ate and How Much					
Comments :					

Date:		Reading Before	Reading 1 hr After	Reading 2 hrs After	Reading 4 hrs After
Which Meal:					
Time Start:					
Time End:					
What I Ate and How Much					
Comments :					

Date:		Reading Before	Reading 1 hr After	Reading 2 hrs After	Reading 4 hrs After
Which Meal:					
Time Start:					
Time End:					
What I Ate and How Much					
Comments :					

Date:		Reading Before	Reading 1 hr After	Reading 2 hrs After	Reading 4 hrs After
Which Meal:					
Time Start:					
Time End:					
What I Ate and How Much					
Comments :					

Date:		Reading Before	Reading 1 hr After	Reading 2 hrs After	Reading 4 hrs After
Which Meal:					
Time Start:					
Time End:					
What I Ate and How Much					
Comments :					

Date:		Reading Before	Reading 1 hr After	Reading 2 hrs After	Reading 4 hrs After
Which Meal:					
Time Start:					
Time End:					
What I Ate and How Much					
Comments :					

Date:		Reading Before	Reading 1 hr After	Reading 2 hrs After	Reading 4 hrs After
Which Meal:					
Time Start:					
Time End:					
What I Ate and How Much					
Comments :					

Date:		Reading Before	Reading 1 hr After	Reading 2 hrs After	Reading 4 hrs After
Which Meal:					
Time Start:					
Time End:					
What I Ate and How Much					
Comments :					

Date:		Reading Before	Reading 1 hr After	Reading 2 hrs After	Reading 4 hrs After
Which Meal:					
Time Start:					
Time End:					
What I Ate and How Much					
Comments :					

Date:		Reading Before	Reading 1 hr After	Reading 2 hrs After	Reading 4 hrs After
Which Meal:					
Time Start:					
Time End:					
What I Ate and How Much					
Comments :					

Date:		Reading Before	Reading 1 hr After	Reading 2 hrs After	Reading 4 hrs After
Which Meal:					
Time Start:					
Time End:					
What I Ate and How Much					
Comments :					

Date:		Reading Before	Reading 1 hr After	Reading 2 hrs After	Reading 4 hrs After
Which Meal:					
Time Start:					
Time End:					
What I Ate and How Much					
Comments:					

Date:		Reading Before	Reading 1 hr After	Reading 2 hrs After	Reading 4 hrs After
Which Meal:					
Time Start:					
Time End:					
What I Ate and How Much					
Comments:					

Date:		Reading Before	Reading 1 hr After	Reading 2 hrs After	Reading 4 hrs After
Which Meal:					
Time Start:					
Time End:					
What I Ate and How Much					
Comments:					

Date:		Reading Before	Reading 1 hr After	Reading 2 hrs After	Reading 4 hrs After
Which Meal:					
Time Start:					
Time End:					
What I Ate and How Much					
Comments :					

Date:		Reading Before	Reading 1 hr After	Reading 2 hrs After	Reading 4 hrs After
Which Meal:					
Time Start:					
Time End:					
What I Ate and How Much					
Comments :					

Date:		Reading Before	Reading 1 hr After	Reading 2 hrs After	Reading 4 hrs After
Which Meal:					
Time Start:					
Time End:					
What I Ate and How Much					
Comments :					

Date:		Reading Before	Reading 1 hr After	Reading 2 hrs After	Reading 4 hrs After
Which Meal:					
Time Start:					
Time End:					
What I Ate and How Much					
Comments :					

Date:		Reading Before	Reading 1 hr After	Reading 2 hrs After	Reading 4 hrs After
Which Meal:					
Time Start:					
Time End:					
What I Ate and How Much					
Comments :					

Date:		Reading Before	Reading 1 hr After	Reading 2 hrs After	Reading 4 hrs After
Which Meal:					
Time Start:					
Time End:					
What I Ate and How Much					
Comments :					

Date:		Reading Before	Reading 1 hr After	Reading 2 hrs After	Reading 4 hrs After
Which Meal:					
Time Start:					
Time End:					
What I Ate and How Much					
Comments:					

Date:		Reading Before	Reading 1 hr After	Reading 2 hrs After	Reading 4 hrs After
Which Meal:					
Time Start:					
Time End:					
What I Ate and How Much					
Comments:					

Date:		Reading Before	Reading 1 hr After	Reading 2 hrs After	Reading 4 hrs After
Which Meal:					
Time Start:					
Time End:					
What I Ate and How Much					
Comments:					

Date:		Reading Before	Reading 1 hr After	Reading 2 hrs After	Reading 4 hrs After
Which Meal:					
Time Start					
Time End:					
What I Ate and How Much					
Comments :					

Date:		Reading Before	Reading 1 hr After	Reading 2 hrs After	Reading 4 hrs After
Which Meal:					
Time Start					
Time End:					
What I Ate and How Much					
Comments :					

Date:		Reading Before	Reading 1 hr After	Reading 2 hrs After	Reading 4 hrs After
Which Meal:					
Time Start:					
Time End:					
What I Ate and How Much					
Comments :					

Date:		Reading Before	Reading 1 hr After	Reading 2 hrs After	Reading 4 hrs After
Which Meal:					
Time Start:					
Time End:					
What I Ate and How Much					
Comments:					

Date:		Reading Before	Reading 1 hr After	Reading 2 hrs After	Reading 4 hrs After
Which Meal:					
Time Start:					
Time End:					
What I Ate and How Much					
Comments:					

Date:		Reading Before	Reading 1 hr After	Reading 2 hrs After	Reading 4 hrs After
Which Meal:					
Time Start:					
Time End:					
What I Ate and How Much					
Comments:					

Date:		Reading Before	Reading 1 hr After	Reading 2 hrs After	Reading 4 hrs After
Which Meal:					
Time Start:					
Time End:					
What I Ate and How Much					
Comments :					

Date:		Reading Before	Reading 1 hr After	Reading 2 hrs After	Reading 4 hrs After
Which Meal:					
Time Start:					
Time End:					
What I Ate and How Much					
Comments :					

Date:		Reading Before	Reading 1 hr After	Reading 2 hrs After	Reading 4 hrs After
Which Meal:					
Time Start:					
Time End:					
What I Ate and How Much					
Comments :					

		Reading Before	Reading 1 hr After	Reading 2 hrs After	Reading 4 hrs After
Date:					
Which Meal:					
Time Start:					
Time End:					
What I Ate and How Much					
Comments :					

		Reading Before	Reading 1 hr After	Reading 2 hrs After	Reading 4 hrs After
Date:					
Which Meal:					
Time Start:					
Time End:					
What I Ate and How Much					
Comments :					

		Reading Before	Reading 1 hr After	Reading 2 hrs After	Reading 4 hrs After
Date:					
Which Meal:					
Time Start:					
Time End:					
What I Ate and How Much					
Comments :					

Date:		Reading Before	Reading 1 hr After	Reading 2 hrs After	Reading 4 hrs After
Which Meal:					
Time Start:					
Time End:					
What I Ate and How Much					
Comments :					

Date:		Reading Before	Reading 1 hr After	Reading 2 hrs After	Reading 4 hrs After
Which Meal:					
Time Start:					
Time End:					
What I Ate and How Much					
Comments :					

Date:		Reading Before	Reading 1 hr After	Reading 2 hrs After	Reading 4 hrs After
Which Meal:					
Time Start:					
Time End:					
What I Ate and How Much					
Comments :					

Date:		Reading Before	Reading 1 hr After	Reading 2 hrs After	Reading 4 hrs After
Which Meal:					
Time Start:					
Time End:					
What I Ate and How Much					
Comments :					

Date:		Reading Before	Reading 1 hr After	Reading 2 hrs After	Reading 4 hrs After
Which Meal:					
Time Start:					
Time End:					
What I Ate and How Much					
Comments :					

Date:		Reading Before	Reading 1 hr After	Reading 2 hrs After	Reading 4 hrs After
Which Meal:					
Time Start:					
Time End:					
What I Ate and How Much					
Comments :					

Date:		Reading Before	Reading 1 hr After	Reading 2 hrs After	Reading 4 hrs After
Which Meal:					
Time Start:					
Time End:					
What I Ate and How Much					
Comments:					

Date:		Reading Before	Reading 1 hr After	Reading 2 hrs After	Reading 4 hrs After
Which Meal:					
Time Start:					
Time End:					
What I Ate and How Much					
Comments:					

Date:		Reading Before	Reading 1 hr After	Reading 2 hrs After	Reading 4 hrs After
Which Meal:					
Time Start:					
Time End:					
What I Ate and How Much					
Comments:					

Date:		Reading Before	Reading 1 hr After	Reading 2 hrs After	Reading 4 hrs After
Which Meal:					
Time Start:					
Time End:					
What I Ate and How Much					
Comments :					

Date:		Reading Before	Reading 1 hr After	Reading 2 hrs After	Reading 4 hrs After
Which Meal:					
Time Start:					
Time End:					
What I Ate and How Much					
Comments :					

Date:		Reading Before	Reading 1 hr After	Reading 2 hrs After	Reading 4 hrs After
Which Meal:					
Time Start:					
Time End:					
What I Ate and How Much					
Comments :					

Date:		Reading Before	Reading 1 hr After	Reading 2 hrs After	Reading 4 hrs After
Which Meal:					
Time Start:					
Time End:					
What I Ate and How Much					
Comments :					

Date:		Reading Before	Reading 1 hr After	Reading 2 hrs After	Reading 4 hrs After
Which Meal:					
Time Start:					
Time End:					
What I Ate and How Much					
Comments :					

Date:		Reading Before	Reading 1 hr After	Reading 2 hrs After	Reading 4 hrs After
Which Meal:					
Time Start:					
Time End:					
What I Ate and How Much					
Comments :					

BOOKS BY Irwin Tyler (Yirmi Tyler)

UNDERSTANDING QUANTUM - Volume 1

The Universe is Made Up of "Stuff"

UNDERSTANDING QUANTUM - Volume 2

The Universe Doesn't Make Any Sense

UNDERSTANDING QUANTUM - Volume 3

The Theory of Everything

POINTS OF HEALTH

The Effectiveness and Safety of Acupuncture and Acupressure

WHY ACUPUNCTURE? - When Conventional Medicine Isn't Working As You Hoped

WHY ACUPRESSURE? - When Conventional Medicine Isn't Working As You Hoped

WHY CHIROPRACTIC? - When Conventional Medicine Isn't Working As You Hoped

WHY HOMEOPATHY? - When Conventional Medicine Isn't Working As You Hoped

THE DIET CHOICE PROGRAM - Beat the Cravings and Enjoy Your Dinner

SO MANY GATES TO THE CITY... A GUIDE FOR THE MODERN PERPLEXED

A Book About Jewish Belief and Understanding, and Making Some Sense Of It

TARGUM AMERICANA - BERESHIT / GENESIS

COLLECTING PAPER MONEY WITH CONFIDENCE

GRADING COINS WITH CONFIDENCE

AMAZON.COM

Selected titles available at:

LULU.COM

CREATESPACE.COM

AHL KAYN PUBLICATIONS WEB SITE

www.ingramcontent.com/pod-product-compliance
Lightning Source LLC
Chambersburg PA
CBHW070133290526
45789CB00005B/2223